TACO DIET REVOLUTION

Lose Weight While Savoring Every Bite

Dr. Raymond F. Bernard

TABLE OF CONTENTS

CHAPTER 1

Introduction - Embracing the Taco Diet

In a world where diet trends come and go like waves on the shore, there's one culinary delight that has withstood the test of time and continues to captivate our taste buds—tacos. In this opening chapter, we embark on a journey that introduces you to the concept of the Taco Diet and lays the foundation for a flavorful and health-conscious adventure.

The Taco's Timeless Allure

Tacos have an enduring appeal that transcends generations and borders. These versatile culinary creations have their origins deeply rooted in Mexican cuisine, but they've evolved into a global sensation, gracing menus from street food vendors to high-end restaurants. From the savory aroma of sizzling meat on a griddle to the colorful medley of toppings that adorn soft or crispy tortillas, tacos are a celebration of flavors, textures, and cultures.

But why tacos, you might ask? What sets them apart from the myriad of other food choices in our world? The answer lies in their simplicity and versatility. Tacos can be as basic or as extravagant as your imagination allows. They can cater to various dietary preferences, from omnivores to vegans. Tacos effortlessly blend tradition with innovation, making them a canvas for culinary creativity.

The Author's Passion for Tacos

Before we dive into the Taco Diet's principles and practices, it's important to understand the author's personal connection to tacos and why they are deeply passionate about this culinary adventure.

The author's journey with tacos began like many others, with a love for the flavors and a curiosity about their potential health benefits. However, what truly ignited their passion was witnessing the transformative power of tacos in their own life. They discovered that tacos could be more than just a delicious treat; they could be the cornerstone of a balanced and sustainable diet.

For the author, tacos became a symbol of joy and balance. They learned to appreciate the beauty of portion control and the art of combining wholesome ingredients in a way that both nourished the body and delighted the senses. Tacos became a daily reminder that healthy eating didn't have to be bland or restrictive. Instead, it could be a celebration of taste, a journey of culinary exploration, and a path to better health.

A Balanced Approach to Healthy Eating

At its core, the Taco Diet is about balance. It's a departure from the restrictive and often unsustainable diet fads that dominate headlines and social media. Instead of shunning entire food groups or obsessively counting calories, the Taco Diet encourages a holistic approach to nutrition.

This approach is grounded in the belief that food should be a source of pleasure and nourishment, not a source of guilt or anxiety. Tacos serve as the perfect embodiment of this philosophy. They invite us to savor the flavors of life while maintaining a sense of equilibrium.

A Journey into the Taco Diet

As we delve deeper into this book, you'll discover that the Taco Diet is not a one-size-fits-all solution. It's not about prescribing rigid meal plans or imposing strict rules. Instead, it's a framework that empowers you to make informed and mindful choices about the food you consume.

Throughout the chapters to come, we'll explore the history of tacos and their cultural significance, learning how they've evolved from humble beginnings to global icons of culinary delight. We'll dissect the art of taco making, offering tips and techniques to elevate your taco game from ordinary to extraordinary.

But this journey isn't just about recipes and cooking methods; it's about understanding the Taco Diet's underlying philosophy. We'll explore the nutritional benefits of key taco ingredients, such as lean proteins, fresh vegetables, and whole grains. We'll debunk common misconceptions about tacos and health, showing you that these delectable creations can indeed be part of a balanced diet.

We'll take you by the hand through the process of crafting healthy taco recipes that cater to different dietary preferences, whether you're a meat lover, a vegetarian, or a dedicated vegan. Each recipe will be thoughtfully designed to strike a harmonious balance between flavor and nutrition, and we'll provide you with calorie counts and portion guidance to make your meal planning easier.

Weekly meal plans will be your roadmap to integrating the Taco Diet into your life. We'll provide you with sample plans that demonstrate how tacos can become a regular and enjoyable part of your diet. You'll receive shopping lists and prep-ahead tips to streamline your meal planning and ensure that it's both convenient and sustainable.

Real-life success stories will inspire you as you read about individuals who have embraced the Taco Diet and achieved their health and wellness goals. These stories are not about extreme transformations but rather about people finding joy and balance in their lives through the simple act of enjoying tacos.

We'll also delve into the practical aspects of sustaining a Taco Diet lifestyle. You'll learn how to navigate dining out, traveling, and handling social situations while staying true to your commitment to healthy eating. Ultimately, we want you to see the Taco Diet not as a temporary fix but as a sustainable way of nourishing your body and soul.

As we conclude this introductory chapter, we invite you to embark on this flavorful journey with an open heart and an adventurous palate. The Taco Diet is not just a diet; it's a celebration of food, culture, and life itself. It's an invitation to savor every bite, to find delight in nourishing your body, and to discover the art of balance through the joy of tacos.

So, let's take that first step together and embrace the Taco Diet as a path to a healthier and more flavorful life.

CHAPTER 2

The Art of Taco Making

In this chapter, we embark on a delightful exploration of the art of taco making. Tacos are more than just a food; they're a culinary tradition deeply rooted in Mexican culture and beloved worldwide. We'll dive into the rich history of tacos, discuss their cultural significance, and unravel the techniques that make crafting the perfect taco a true art form.

The Origins of Tacos

To truly appreciate the art of taco making, it's essential to understand where tacos come from. Tacos have a long and storied history that dates back centuries, rooted in the heart of Mexico. The word "taco" itself is believed to have originated from the Nahuatl language, spoken by the Aztecs, and it referred to a small piece of paper used to wrap around food.

Historians suggest that the earliest tacos were simple, with indigenous people in Mexico using soft tortillas made from corn or other locally available grains to scoop up small portions of various fillings, including beans, insects, and small game. These early tacos were a practical and portable way to enjoy a quick meal.

As Spanish conquistadors arrived in the Americas, they encountered indigenous people enjoying these tortilla-wrapped delights. The Spanish brought with them new ingredients like beef, pork, and dairy, which were quickly incorporated into the taco-making tradition. Over time, the taco evolved, becoming a fusion of indigenous and European flavors.

Cultural Significance of Tacos

Tacos have transcended their humble origins to become a symbol of Mexican cuisine and culture. They are a cornerstone of Mexican street food, where vendors craft tacos with skill and passion, often specializing in a particular type of taco, such as al pastor, carnitas, or barbacoa.

Tacos also play a central role in Mexican celebrations and traditions. They are a staple at fiestas, weddings, and other festive gatherings. The act of making and sharing tacos is an expression of hospitality and community, bringing people together around a communal table.

Beyond Mexico, tacos have become a global phenomenon. They've been embraced and adapted by countless cultures, each putting its unique spin on these delectable creations. From Korean BBQ tacos to Indian-inspired curry tacos, the possibilities are endless, highlighting the universal appeal of this versatile dish.

The Taco-Making Toolkit

Before we dive into the techniques of taco making, let's gather our tools. While you don't need a fancy kitchen setup to make delicious tacos, a few key items can greatly enhance your taco-making experience:

1. **Tortillas:** The foundation of any taco is the tortilla. You can choose between soft flour tortillas or traditional corn tortillas. Opt for high-quality, fresh tortillas whenever possible, as they make a significant difference in taste and texture.

2. **Proteins:** Tacos can feature a variety of proteins, from classic options like beef,

chicken, and pork to vegetarian and vegan alternatives like tofu, tempeh, or plant-based meat substitutes. Select proteins that align with your dietary preferences and nutritional goals.

3. **Fresh Ingredients:** Tacos are an excellent way to incorporate fresh vegetables into your diet. Consider options like lettuce, tomatoes, onions, bell peppers, avocados, and cilantro. These not only add vibrant colors but also provide essential nutrients.

4. **Cheese:** If you enjoy dairy, cheese can be a delightful addition to your tacos. Common choices include cheddar, Monterey Jack, or crumbly queso fresco. Grated or crumbled, cheese adds creaminess and depth of flavor.

5. **Sauces and Salsas:** Elevate your tacos with a selection of sauces and salsas. From mild and tangy to spicy and smoky, there are countless options to choose from. Consider classics like salsa verde, pico de gallo, or a creamy chipotle sauce.

6. **Spices and Seasonings:** A well-stocked spice cabinet is essential for flavoring your taco fillings. Common seasonings include cumin, chili powder, paprika, garlic powder, and oregano. Experiment with combinations to create your signature taco seasoning.

7. **Cooking Equipment:** Depending on your protein choice, you may need a skillet, grill, or oven for cooking. Having a good-quality non-stick pan or a cast-iron skillet can be particularly useful for

achieving that perfect sear on your meat or tofu.

Now that we've assembled our taco-making toolkit, let's explore the art of crafting delicious tacos:

Techniques for Perfect Tacos

1. **Properly Heating Tortillas:** Warm tortillas are crucial for a great taco experience. You can heat them in a dry skillet, microwave, or on a hot griddle for a short time until they're pliable and slightly toasted. Keep them warm in a clean kitchen towel or

tortilla warmer to maintain their temperature.

2. **Choosing and Preparing Proteins:** Whether you're cooking meat, poultry, seafood, or plant-based proteins, aim for even cooking and flavorful results. Marinate proteins in your chosen seasonings for at least 15 minutes to infuse them with flavor. When cooking, avoid overcrowding the pan to ensure proper searing.

3. **Layering Ingredients:** The order of ingredient placement matters. Start

with proteins, followed by fresh vegetables and cheese. This layering helps the cheese melt and the vegetables stay crisp. Finish with a drizzle of sauce or salsa for a burst of flavor.

4. **Balancing Flavors and Textures:** A great taco balances flavors and textures. Consider contrasts like spicy and creamy, crunchy and tender, and sweet and savory. For example, pair spicy salsa with cool avocado, or tender carnitas with crisp pickled onions.

5. **Garnishing and Presentation:** Don't underestimate the power of garnishes. Fresh herbs like cilantro, a squeeze of lime, or a sprinkle of crumbled cheese can elevate your taco's appearance and taste.

6. **Customization:** Tacos are inherently customizable. Invite your guests or family members to build their own tacos with a variety of fillings, sauces, and toppings. It's a fun and interactive way to enjoy a meal together.

7. **Exploring Taco Styles:** Tacos come in various styles, including street tacos, hard-shell tacos, and even dessert tacos. Experiment with different styles to discover your favorites and keep your taco repertoire exciting.

In this chapter, we've scratched the surface of the art of taco making. Tacos are more than just a meal; they are a canvas for culinary creativity, a reflection of cultural diversity, and a testament to the joy of communal dining. As we proceed through this book, you'll learn how to apply these techniques to create healthy and delicious taco recipes that align with the Taco Diet's principles of balance and flavor. So, grab your tortillas, assemble your ingredients, and let's continue our flavorful journey into the world of the Taco Diet.

CHAPTER 3

The Taco Diet Philosophy

In this chapter, we delve deep into the heart and soul of the Taco Diet. Beyond the delicious recipes and the art of taco making, it's essential to understand the guiding principles and philosophy that make this diet not just a passing trend but a sustainable and enjoyable approach to healthy eating.

Balanced and Sustainable Nutrition

At its core, the Taco Diet promotes a philosophy of balanced and sustainable nutrition. It rejects the notion that healthy eating should be synonymous with deprivation or rigid restrictions. Instead, it encourages you to embrace food as a source of nourishment and pleasure while maintaining a sense of equilibrium.

This philosophy is grounded in the belief that a balanced diet can lead to better overall health and well-being. Rather than fixating on the latest diet trends or extreme eating plans, the Taco Diet encourages you to focus on a diverse range of foods that provide essential nutrients, vitamins, and minerals.

Tacos as a Perfect Vessel for Balance

Tacos are the ideal embodiment of the Taco Diet philosophy. They are a culinary canvas where you can effortlessly create balanced and satisfying meals. Consider the components of a classic taco:

1. **Proteins:** Tacos can feature lean proteins such as grilled chicken, turkey, or fish, providing a source of

essential amino acids for muscle health and overall energy.

2. **Vegetables:** Fresh vegetables like lettuce, tomatoes, onions, and bell peppers add color and texture to your tacos, while also supplying vitamins, fiber, and antioxidants.

3. **Whole Grains:** Corn tortillas, a common choice for traditional tacos, offer whole grains that provide complex carbohydrates for sustained energy.

4. **Dairy:** If you enjoy dairy, options like cheese or

yogurt-based sauces contribute calcium and protein.

5. **Healthy Fats:** Avocado, a popular taco ingredient, contains healthy monounsaturated fats that support heart health.

6. **Flavorful Spices:** The seasonings used in taco recipes, such as cumin, chili powder, and garlic, not only enhance taste but can also have potential health benefits.

By carefully selecting and combining these elements in your

tacos, you create a harmonious meal that satisfies your palate while also meeting your nutritional needs. The Taco Diet teaches you to appreciate the inherent balance in this culinary art form.

Dismantling Myths about Tacos and Health

One of the key goals of the Taco Diet is to dismantle common misconceptions about tacos and their role in a healthy diet. Tacos have often been unfairly labeled as unhealthy, thanks in part to the fast-food versions that are loaded with excess calories, saturated fats, and sodium.

However, it's important to recognize that tacos, like any other food, can be made in a way that aligns with your health and dietary goals. When prepared thoughtfully, tacos can be both nutritious and delicious.

Here are some myths about tacos and their associated truths:

Myth 1: Tacos are always high in calories and unhealthy.

- Truth: Tacos' calorie content varies greatly depending on their ingredients and portion sizes. The Taco Diet emphasizes portion control and nutrient-dense fillings to keep calories in check.

Myth 2: Tacos are not suitable for a balanced diet.

- Truth: Tacos can be a part of a balanced diet when made with fresh ingredients, lean proteins, and plenty of vegetables. They offer a balanced combination of macronutrients.

Myth 3: Tacos are inherently greasy and fattening.

- Truth: Tacos do not have to be greasy or fattening. Grilled or baked proteins, minimal oil usage, and avocado-based sauces are all healthier alternatives.

Myth 4: Tacos are not suitable for vegetarians or vegans.

- Truth: Tacos are incredibly versatile and can be adapted to suit various dietary preferences. Plant-based proteins like tofu, beans, or tempeh make excellent taco fillings.

By debunking these myths, the Taco Diet encourages you to approach tacos with an open mind and a discerning eye, recognizing that they can be part of a balanced and health-conscious diet.

The Joy of Eating Mindfully

Mindful eating is a cornerstone of the Taco Diet philosophy. It's about savoring each bite, being present in the moment, and paying attention to the flavors and textures of your food. When you eat mindfully, you're less likely to overindulge, and you can better appreciate the nuances of your meal.

Tacos provide an excellent opportunity for mindful eating. As you assemble your taco, take a moment to appreciate the vibrant colors, the enticing aromas, and the variety of textures. When you take that first bite, savor the combination of flavors and the sensation of each ingredient.

Mindful eating isn't just about enjoying your meal; it's also about listening to your body's hunger and fullness cues. By tuning in to your body's signals, you can avoid overeating and better understand your dietary needs.

The Taco Diet as a Lifestyle Choice

Ultimately, the Taco Diet isn't just a temporary diet plan; it's a lifestyle choice. It's a way of approaching food that emphasizes balance, sustainability, and pleasure. It encourages you to find joy in your food choices, to celebrate the act of cooking and sharing meals, and to make thoughtful decisions about what you eat.

Throughout this book, you'll find practical guidance on how to apply the Taco Diet philosophy to your daily life. We'll provide you with delicious and balanced taco recipes that align with these principles, helping you discover how tacos can be a regular and enjoyable part of your diet.

As we proceed through the chapters, you'll learn more about crafting healthy taco recipes, planning balanced meals, and sustaining the Taco Diet in various real-life situations. Together, we'll embark on a flavorful journey that goes beyond dieting and embraces a lifelong commitment to nourishing your body and soul through the joy of tacos. So, let's continue this exploration of the

Taco Diet philosophy, finding the
perfect blend of flavor and balance
in every taco bite.

CHAPTER 4

Crafting Healthy Taco Recipes

In this chapter, we'll dive deep into the heart of the Taco Diet by exploring the creative and flavorful world of healthy taco recipes. Tacos are not only delicious but also incredibly versatile, making them the perfect vessel for crafting balanced and nutritious meals that align with the principles of the Taco Diet.

Taco Recipes: Beyond the Basics

Tacos come in a wide variety of styles and flavors, which means there's a taco recipe for everyone, regardless of dietary preferences. The Taco Diet embraces this diversity and encourages you to explore different combinations of ingredients to create tacos that suit your taste and nutritional needs.

Here are some essential elements of crafting healthy taco recipes:

1. **Lean Proteins:** Choose proteins that are lean and rich in nutrients. Options like grilled chicken, turkey, fish, shrimp, lean beef, and

ground turkey are excellent choices. For plant-based diets, consider tofu, tempeh, or legumes like black beans or lentils.

2. **Fresh Vegetables:** Load up your tacos with a variety of fresh vegetables to add color, crunch, and essential nutrients. Tomatoes, lettuce, bell peppers, onions, and avocados are classic taco toppings. Experiment with others like spinach, kale, or radishes for added flavor and nutrition.

3. **Whole Grains:** Traditional tacos often use corn tortillas,

which offer whole grains. If you prefer flour tortillas, look for whole-grain options. You can also explore alternatives like lettuce wraps or whole-grain pita pockets for a lower-carb option.

4. **Healthy Fats:** Incorporate healthy fats into your tacos for flavor and satiety. Avocado slices, guacamole, or a drizzle of olive oil-based dressing can provide the desirable healthy fat content.

5. **Flavorful Spices:** Experiment with a variety of spices to season your taco

fillings. Common taco seasonings include cumin, chili powder, paprika, garlic powder, and oregano. These not only enhance taste but also offer potential health benefits.

6. **Sauces and Salsas:** Elevate the flavor of your tacos with a selection of sauces and salsas. From mild and tangy to spicy and smoky, there are countless options to choose from. Consider classics like salsa verde, pico de gallo, or a creamy chipotle sauce.

Balancing Flavors and Nutrients

A crucial aspect of crafting healthy taco recipes is achieving a balance of flavors and nutrients. Healthy tacos should be both delicious and nutritionally well-rounded. Here's how you can achieve this balance:

1. **Protein and Vegetables:** Ensure that your tacos include a generous portion of lean protein and a variety of fresh vegetables. This combination provides essential nutrients and keeps you feeling satisfied.

2. **Complex Carbohydrates:**
   If you're using tortillas, opt
   for whole-grain versions to
   add complex carbohydrates
   to your meal. These provide
   sustained energy and fiber to
   keep you full.

3. **Healthy Fats:** Incorporate
   healthy fats, such as those
   found in avocados or olive
   oil-based dressings, to
   enhance the flavor and
   satiety of your tacos.

4. **Flavorful Seasonings:**
   Use a mix of spices to create
   a flavorful taco filling. This
   not only makes your tacos
   tastier but can also have

potential health benefits, depending on the spices used.

5. **Sauces and Salsas:** Experiment with sauces and salsas to add zing to your tacos. These condiments can transform a simple taco into a flavor-packed delight. Be mindful of portion sizes, especially if they are calorie-dense.

Sample Healthy Taco Recipes

Let's explore some sample healthy taco recipes that showcase the Taco Diet's principles of balance and flavor:

1. **Grilled Chicken and Avocado Tacos**

- Lean protein: Grilled chicken breast seasoned with a blend of cumin, paprika, and garlic powder.
- Fresh vegetables: Sliced tomatoes, diced onions, and shredded lettuce.
- Healthy fats: Slices of creamy avocado.
- Whole grains: Soft whole-grain corn tortillas.
- Flavorful salsa: Freshly made pico de gallo with diced tomatoes, onions,

cilantro, and a squeeze of lime.

2. Spicy Black Bean and Vegetable Tacos

- Plant-based protein: Spiced black beans cooked with chili powder and cumin.
- Fresh vegetables: Sautéed bell peppers, onions, and spinach.
- Whole grains: Whole-grain flour tortillas or lettuce wraps.
- Healthy fats: A dollop of guacamole.

- Flavorful spices: A pinch of smoked paprika and cayenne for extra kick.

3. Grilled Shrimp and Mango Salsa Tacos

- Lean protein: Grilled shrimp marinated in a lime and cilantro dressing.
- Fresh vegetables and fruits: A refreshing mango salsa with diced mangoes, red onions, cilantro, and jalapeños.
- Whole grains: Soft corn tortillas.
- Healthy fats: A drizzle of olive oil-based dressing.

- Flavorful spices: A hint of ground coriander and a dash of cayenne pepper for complexity.

4. Veggie Delight Lettuce Wrap Tacos

- Plant-based protein: Sautéed mushrooms, bell peppers, and onions seasoned with a mix of herbs and spices.

- Fresh vegetables: Shredded cabbage, diced tomatoes, and sliced avocado.

- Whole grains: Large lettuce leaves as wraps.

- Healthy fats: A sprinkle of crushed nuts for crunch and healthy fats.
- Flavorful sauces: A tangy Greek yogurt-based dressing.

These sample recipes demonstrate the diversity and creativity that healthy tacos offer. Whether you prefer classic flavors, crave a bit of spice, or enjoy the sweetness of fruits, there's a healthy taco recipe for you.

Portion Control and Mindful Eating

While crafting healthy taco recipes is important, it's equally crucial to practice portion control and mindful eating. Tacos can be deceptively easy to overindulge in, especially when they're delicious.

Here are some tips for portion control and mindful eating with tacos:

1. **Use Smaller Tortillas:** Opt for smaller tortillas to help control portion sizes. Mini tortillas or taco-sized tortillas can make a big difference in calorie intake.

2. **Fill Moderately:** Avoid overstuffing your tacos.

Balance the amount of filling with the size of the tortilla to keep portions reasonable.

3. **Include Fiber:** Ensure your tacos contain fiber-rich ingredients like vegetables and whole grains. Fiber helps promote feelings of fullness and satisfaction.

4. **Eat Mindfully:** Take your time to savor each bite. Put down your taco between bites, chew slowly, and appreciate the flavors and textures.

5. **Listen to Your Body:** Pay attention to your body's hunger and fullness cues.

Stop eating when you're satisfied, not overly full.

Experimenting and Customization

The beauty of healthy taco recipes is their flexibility. Feel free to experiment with different ingredients, seasonings, and styles of tacos to find what suits your taste and nutritional goals. Tacos can be tailored to various dietary preferences, from omnivorous to vegetarian and vegan.

Customization is also a fun aspect of taco preparation. Consider setting up a taco bar for family and friends, allowing everyone to assemble their tacos with their preferred fillings and toppings. It's an interactive and enjoyable way to share a meal together.

In conclusion, chapter 4 takes us into the heart of the Taco Diet by exploring the wonderful world of healthy taco recipes. Tacos are more than just a meal; they are a canvas for culinary creativity, a reflection of cultural diversity, and a testament to the joy of communal dining. By crafting balanced and nutritious tacos that align with the Taco Diet's principles, you not only nourish your body but also delight your taste buds. As we continue our flavorful journey, you'll discover even more recipes and tips to help you embrace the Taco Diet as a delicious and sustainable approach to healthy eating. So, let's keep exploring the art of crafting healthy taco recipes, one flavorful bite at a time.

CHAPTER 5

Weekly Taco Meal Plans

In this chapter, we will delve into the practical side of the Taco Diet by providing you with sample weekly taco meal plans. These meal plans are designed to help you seamlessly incorporate tacos into your regular eating routine while adhering to the Taco Diet's principles of balance, flavor, and nutrition.

The Importance of Meal Planning

Meal planning is a cornerstone of successful and sustainable healthy eating. It empowers you to make mindful choices about your food, ensures that you have nutritious options readily available, and can save you time and money. By crafting weekly taco meal plans, you'll not only simplify your daily food decisions but also enjoy the convenience of having a well-balanced and flavorful meal waiting for you.

Balancing Macronutrients

The Taco Diet encourages balance in your meals, and that includes macronutrients – carbohydrates, proteins, and fats. A well-balanced meal helps you feel satisfied, maintains stable energy levels, and provides the essential nutrients your body needs. Here's how we incorporate this balance into the meal plans:

1. **Protein:** Each meal plan includes a variety of proteins, both animal and plant-based, to ensure you get a diverse range of amino acids.

2. **Carbohydrates:** We incorporate whole grains, primarily through whole-grain tortillas or wraps, to provide complex carbohydrates for sustained energy.

3. **Fats:** Healthy fats, often from avocado or olive oil-based dressings, are included to enhance flavor and satiety.

4. **Fiber:** Vegetables and legumes are key components of these meal plans, providing fiber that aids in digestion and keeps you feeling full.

5. **Portion Control:** We emphasize portion control to help you manage calorie intake and prevent overeating.

Sample Weekly Taco Meal Plans

Let's explore some sample weekly taco meal plans that showcase how tacos can be an integral part of your diet while following the Taco Diet's principles.

Meal Plan 1: Balanced Week

Day 1: Classic Chicken Tacos

- Lunch: Grilled chicken tacos with lettuce, tomato, and a light yogurt-based sauce.
- Dinner: Baked fish tacos with slaw and avocado slices.

Day 2: Vegetarian Delight

- Lunch: Black bean and corn tacos with salsa and a side of mixed greens.
- Dinner: Grilled vegetable and tofu tacos with a drizzle of balsamic glaze.

Day 3: Lean Protein Fiesta

- Lunch: Ground turkey tacos with sautéed bell peppers and onions.
- Dinner: Shrimp tacos with mango salsa and a side of quinoa salad.

Day 4: Meatless Monday

- Lunch: Lentil and mushroom tacos with

spinach and a tahini dressing.

- Dinner: Vegan chickpea and sweet potato tacos with a lime-cilantro sauce.

Day 5: Fusion Friday

- Lunch: Korean BBQ beef tacos with kimchi and pickled cucumbers.
- Dinner: Thai-inspired chicken satay tacos with peanut sauce.

Day 6: Weekend Brunch Special

- Brunch: Breakfast tacos with scrambled eggs, sautéed spinach, and salsa.

- Dinner: Grilled steak tacos with chimichurri sauce and a side of roasted sweet potatoes.

Day 7: Fiesta Finale

- Lunch: Carnitas tacos with pickled red onions and jalapeños.
- Dinner: Grilled portobello mushroom tacos with avocado crema.

Meal Plan 2: Quick and Easy Week

Day 1: Taco Salad Night

- Lunch: Taco salad with ground chicken, black beans, and a zesty vinaigrette.
- Dinner: Turkey and avocado wrap in a whole-grain tortilla.

Day 2: Sheet Pan Supper

- Lunch: Vegetarian roasted vegetable tacos with feta and a lemon-tahini drizzle.
- Dinner: Sheet pan shrimp fajita tacos with bell peppers and onions.

Day 3: Busy Day Tacos

- Lunch: Make-ahead turkey taco bowl with salsa and Greek yogurt.
- Dinner: Quick chicken and avocado tacos with pre-made slaw.

Day 4: Vegan Vibes

- Lunch: Vegan black bean and quinoa tacos with cilantro-lime dressing.
- Dinner: Tempeh taco lettuce wraps with a spicy sriracha sauce.

Day 5: Taco Night Out

- Lunch: Leftover tacos from dinner out – choose lean

protein and load up on veggies.

- Dinner: Homemade fish tacos with mango salsa and a side of brown rice.

Day 6: Breakfast for Dinner

- Brunch: Breakfast tacos with scrambled eggs, spinach, and salsa.
- Dinner: Grilled steak tacos with a side of sautéed asparagus.

Day 7: Taco Pizza Night

- Lunch: Taco-inspired pizza with ground turkey, bell

peppers, and a whole-grain crust.

- Dinner: Shrimp and avocado tacos with a side salad.

Meal Plan 3: Vegetarian Delights

Day 1: Meatless Monday Fiesta

- Lunch: Vegan chickpea and sweet potato tacos with a lime-cilantro sauce.
- Dinner: Portobello mushroom and black bean tacos with avocado crema.

Day 2: Taco Salad Bowl

- Lunch: Taco salad bowl with quinoa, grilled tofu, and a spicy sriracha dressing.
- Dinner: Baked falafel and hummus wrap in a whole-grain tortilla.

Day 3: Lentil and Spinach Tacos

- Lunch: Lentil and mushroom tacos with spinach and a tahini dressing.
- Dinner: Vegetable stir-fry tofu tacos with hoisin sauce.

Day 4: Fusion Flavors

- Lunch: Thai-inspired peanut tofu tacos with pickled cucumber.
- Dinner: Korean BBQ tempeh tacos with kimchi.

Day 5: Brunch Tacos

- Brunch: Breakfast tacos with scrambled eggs, sautéed spinach, and salsa.
- Dinner: Vegan cauliflower and chickpea tacos with a lemon-tahini drizzle.

Day 6: Sheet Pan Supper

- Lunch: Vegan roasted vegetable tacos with a balsamic glaze.

- Dinner: Sheet pan halloumi cheese and vegetable tacos.

Day 7: Taco Pizza Night

- Lunch: Taco-inspired pizza with black beans, bell peppers, and a whole-grain crust.
- Dinner: Vegan tempeh and avocado tacos with a side salad.

These sample weekly meal plans provide you with a diverse array of taco options while maintaining a balanced approach to nutrition. Feel free to mix and match recipes to suit your preferences and dietary needs.

Additional Tips for Successful Meal Planning

1. **Prep Ahead:** Take advantage of meal prep by preparing ingredients in advance. Chop vegetables, marinate proteins, and make sauces so that assembling your tacos is quick and easy during the week.

2. **Variety is Key:** Rotate ingredients and flavors to keep your meals exciting and prevent dietary boredom. Experiment with different

protein sources, seasonings, and vegetables.

3. **Mindful Eating:** Remember to practice mindful eating during your meals. Pay attention to portion sizes, savor each bite, and listen to your body's hunger and fullness cues.

4. **Grocery List:** Create a grocery list based on your meal plan to ensure you have all the necessary ingredients on hand. This can help reduce food waste and save you time during the week.

5. **Taco Bar Fun:** Host a taco night with friends or family where everyone can build their tacos with a variety of fillings and toppings. It's a fun and interactive way to enjoy tacos together.

6. **Experiment and Adapt:** Don't be afraid to adapt the meal plans to your dietary preferences and requirements. Whether you're vegetarian, vegan, or omnivorous, there are endless taco possibilities to explore.

In conclusion, chapter 5 offers you a practical guide to incorporating tacos into your weekly meal plans. Tacos are not only delicious but also versatile and can be adapted to various dietary preferences. By following these meal plans and tips, you'll discover how tacos can be a delightful and nutritious addition to your regular diet, aligning perfectly with the Taco Diet's philosophy of balance and flavor. So, let's continue our journey through the world of tacos, one delicious bite at a time, as we move forward in this book.

CHAPTER 6

Dining Out and Traveling on the Taco Diet

In this chapter, we'll tackle a common challenge faced by many when trying to maintain a healthy eating plan: dining out and traveling. The Taco Diet isn't just about what you eat at home; it's a lifestyle that should be sustainable in various situations. Whether you're dining at a restaurant or exploring new places, we'll explore how to stay true to the Taco Diet's principles of balance and flavor while enjoying meals outside of your home.

The Challenge of Dining Out

Eating out at restaurants can pose a challenge to those following specific dietary plans, but with the right strategies, it can be an enjoyable experience that aligns with the Taco Diet.

1. **Research Ahead:** Before heading to a restaurant, look up the menu online. Many restaurants provide their menu online, along with nutritional information. This allows you to

make informed choices and plan your meal in advance.

2. Choose Wisely: When browsing the menu, focus on options that align with the Taco Diet's principles. Look for lean protein options, plenty of vegetables, and whole-grain or lower-carb alternatives like whole-grain tortillas or lettuce wraps.

3. Ask for Modifications: Don't be afraid to ask your server for modifications to suit your preferences and dietary needs. For example, request grilled instead of fried, or ask for dressings and sauces on the side.

4. Mindful Eating: Practice mindful eating when dining out. Pay attention to portion sizes and stop eating when you're satisfied, not when your plate is empty.

5. Share and Split: Consider sharing dishes with a dining partner or splitting a meal if portions are large. This not only helps with portion control but also encourages variety.

6. Be Wary of Extras: Be cautious of extras that can add extra calories, such as appetizers, bread baskets, and sugary beverages. Opt for healthier appetizers like a salad or broth-based soup.

7. Enjoy the Experience: Dining out is not just about the food; it's also about the experience. Savor each bite, enjoy the company of your dining companions, and appreciate the ambiance of the restaurant.

Traveling on the Taco Diet

Traveling often presents unique challenges when it comes to maintaining a specific eating plan, but it's entirely possible to stay true to the Taco Diet while exploring new destinations.

1. **Plan Ahead:** Research restaurants and food options at your travel destination. Identify places that offer balanced and flavorful meals. Apps and websites can be helpful resources for finding restaurants that align with your dietary preferences.

2. **Pack Smart:** If you have specific dietary requirements, consider packing some snacks or portable, non-perishable foods that align with the Taco Diet. This ensures you have nutritious options on hand if healthy choices are limited.

3. Explore Local Cuisine: Embrace the opportunity to explore the local cuisine at your destination. Look for dishes that incorporate fresh ingredients, lean proteins, and vegetables, as these often align with the Taco Diet.

4. Opt for Balance: When dining out while traveling, aim for balance in your meals. Choose dishes that include a variety of food groups, and avoid overindulging in heavy or rich foods.

5. Practice Portion Control: Portions can vary widely from one place to another. If you find that portions are large, consider sharing a meal with a travel companion or asking for a to-go container to enjoy the leftovers later.

6. Stay Hydrated: Don't forget to stay hydrated while traveling. Carry a reusable water bottle and drink plenty of water throughout the day. Sometimes thirst is mistaken for hunger.

7. Be Flexible: While it's important to stay true to the Taco Diet's principles, be flexible when traveling. You may not always find the exact options you're accustomed to, and that's okay.

Adapt and make the healthiest choices available to you.

Taco Diet-Friendly Dining Out Strategies

Now, let's explore some specific strategies for dining out while following the Taco Diet:

1. Mexican Restaurants: Mexican restaurants can be a Taco Diet-friendly choice. Look for options like grilled chicken or shrimp tacos with lots of fresh veggies. Choose corn tortillas over flour for a whole-grain option.

2. Salad Bars: Salad bars offer a plethora of fresh vegetables, lean proteins, and toppings. Create your taco-inspired salad by loading up on greens, adding grilled chicken or beans, and topping it with salsa and a dollop of Greek yogurt or a light dressing.

3. Asian Cuisine: Many Asian cuisines offer balanced options. Consider dishes like stir-fried tofu or chicken with vegetables. Opt for brown rice or whole-grain noodles when available.

4. Mediterranean Restaurants: Mediterranean cuisine often includes grilled proteins, fresh vegetables, and flavorful seasonings. Look for dishes like grilled kebabs or falafel wraps with lots of veggies and hummus.

5. Seafood Restaurants: Seafood restaurants can provide excellent choices for the Taco Diet. Order grilled fish tacos with a side of coleslaw and skip the fried options.

6. Build-Your-Own Tacos: Some restaurants allow you to build your tacos, giving you control over the ingredients. Select lean proteins, whole-grain tortillas, and plenty of vegetables.

7. Sushi Restaurants: While sushi is generally a healthy option, be mindful of portion sizes and opt for rolls that include plenty of vegetables and lean proteins like salmon or tuna.

8. Veggie-Centric Restaurants: If you come across a veggie-centric or plant-based restaurant, explore their menu for creative and nutritious taco-inspired dishes featuring plant-based proteins like tofu, tempeh, or legumes.

Eating on the Go

For those moments when you're on the go and need a quick and healthy meal, consider these options:

1. **Salad Chains:** Many salad chains offer customizable salads and grain bowls where you can create a taco-inspired dish with your favorite ingredients.

2. **Fast-Casual Mexican Chains:** Some fast-casual Mexican chains provide healthier options, including grilled protein choices, brown rice, and whole-grain tortillas.

3. Sandwich Shops: Look for sandwich shops that offer wraps or flatbreads as a healthy and portable option. Fill them with lean proteins and plenty of veggies.

4. Convenience Stores: In a pinch, convenience stores often stock healthier options like pre-packaged salads, yogurt, or fresh fruit. These can be a nutritious snack or meal when you're traveling.

5. Airport Eateries: Airports are becoming increasingly health-conscious in their dining options. Seek out restaurants that offer salads, grain bowls, or protein-rich meals.

Staying True to the Taco Diet

While dining out and traveling can present challenges, they should not deter you from following the Taco Diet's principles of balance and flavor. The key is to be prepared, make informed choices, and adapt when necessary. Remember that the Taco Diet is a flexible and sustainable approach to healthy eating that can be maintained in various situations.

By planning ahead, practicing portion control, and seeking out balanced options, you can enjoy dining out and traveling while staying true to the Taco Diet. Embrace the opportunity to explore new flavors and cuisines, and savor the experience of sharing meals with others, whether you're at home or on the road.

In conclusion, chapter 6 equips you with practical strategies for dining out and traveling while adhering to the Taco Diet. The Taco Diet isn't about deprivation; it's about making mindful and delicious choices that align with your health and taste preferences, no matter where your culinary adventures take you. So, let's continue our journey, exploring the world of tacos while maintaining balance and flavor in every dining experience.

CONCLUSION

In conclusion, the Taco Diet offers a flavorful and balanced approach to healthy eating that celebrates the joy of food while nourishing your body. Throughout this book, we've explored the philosophy of the Taco Diet, crafting healthy taco recipes, planning weekly meal plans, and navigating dining out and traveling while staying true to this lifestyle.

The Taco Diet encourages you to embrace food as more than just sustenance; it's an art form, a means of connection, and a source of pleasure. Tacos, with their versatility and potential for creativity, are the perfect embodiment of this philosophy. They can be tailored to suit various dietary preferences, making them accessible to anyone on a journey toward better health.

By following the principles of balance, flavor, and mindful eating, you can enjoy the Taco Diet as a sustainable and enjoyable lifestyle. Whether you're preparing tacos at home, dining out with friends, or exploring new cuisines while traveling, the Taco Diet empowers you to make informed choices that honor both your well-being and your taste buds.

As you continue your flavorful journey with the Taco Diet, remember that it's not about perfection but about finding harmony in your food choices. It's about savoring each bite, appreciating the colors and textures, and listening to your body's cues. With the Taco Diet, you can nourish your body, satisfy your palate, and celebrate the delightful world of tacos while embracing a lifelong commitment to health and happiness.

So, embark on this flavorful adventure, explore new ingredients and flavors, and relish the experience of crafting and sharing delicious, balanced tacos with friends and loved ones. The Taco Diet is not just a diet; it's a celebration of food, life, and well-being, and it's yours to enjoy.